Essential Oils for Problem Skin:
50 Recipes that Heal Widespread Skin Issues

Table Of Content

Introduction..6

Chapter 1. Essential Oils...7

Chapter 2. Essential Oils Vs. Pharmaceuticals..14

Chapter 3. Collection of Essential Oil Based Skin and Hair Treatments.............16

1. Wood Violet (Viola odorata)...16

2. Bitter Orange (Citrus aurantium)...16

3. Atlas Cedar (Cedar atlantica)...16

4. Cade Juniper (Juniperus oxycedrus)...17

5. Roman chamomile (Chamaemelu m nobile)...17

6. Niaouli (melaleuca quinquen-ervia)..17

7. Tea Tree (Melaleuca alternifolia)...17

8. Helichrysum (Helichrysum)..18

9. Laudanum (Cistus ladaniferus)...18

10. Wild Carrot (daucus carota)...18

11. Lovage (Levisticum officinale)...19

12. Holy Basil (Ocimum sanctum)..19

13. Mandarin (citrus reticulata var. mandarin)..19

14. Sweet Fennel (Foeniculum vulgare var. Dulce)..19

15. Ginger (Zingiber officinalis)...20

16. Ylang-Ylang (Cananga odorata)...20

17. Rosemary camphor (Rosmarinus officinalis cam-phoriferum)......................20

18. Patchouli (Pogostemon cablin)...21

19. Lemon verbena (Lippia citriodora)...21

20. Grapefruit (Citrus paradisii)...21

21. Lime (citrus aurantifolia)..22

22. Lemon (citrus limonum)...22

23. Damask rose (Rosa damascena)..23

24. Neroli (Citrus aurantium)...23

25. Myrtle Green (Myrtus communis cineoliferum)...23

26. Lemon Balm (Melissa officinalis)..24

27. Jasmine (Jasminum grandiflorum) 24

28. Turmeric (Curcuma longa) 24

29. Geranium Rosat (pelargonium asperum)...24

30. Tansy (tanacetum annuum)..25

Chapter 4. Bonus Recipe Collection! 26

31. Vanilla (vanilla planifolia)..26

32. Frankincense or Olibanum (boswellia carterii) 26

33. Garden Angelica (Angelica archangelica)..26

34. Essential Oil Blend Body Powder 27

35. Natural and Pure Skin Toner 27

36. Essential Oil Treatment for Psoriasis: 27

37. Recipe for Treating Oily Hair:..28

38. Essential Oil Blend for Treating Dandruff 29

39. Dull Skin Essential Oil Treatment..29

40. Skin Softening and Healing Recipe..30

41. Muscle Relief Essential Oil Massage 30

42. Essential Oil Massage for Over Exerted Muscles: 30

43. Essential Oil Blend for Muscle Cramps: 31

44. Simple Bruise Oil: 31

45. Massage Oil for Rheumatism: 32

46. Body Butter for Varicose Veins: 33

47. Body Scrub for Sensitive Skin:...33

48. Body Scrub for Oily Skin: 34

49. Body Scrub for Skin with Eczema...34

50. Stretch Mark Serum:...35

Conclusion 36

FREE Bonus Reminder...37

Introduction

I would like to thank and congratulate you for downloading "Essential Oils for Problem Skin: 30 Recipes that Heal Widespread Skin Issues". You will enjoy using these simple but effective recipes that will help to heal and revive your skin with the help of essential oils.

More and more people are seeking skin treatments that are not loaded with artificial ingredients and chemicals that tend to do more harm than good. The more natural products are the less bad side effects they are going to have on your skin. Using essential oil based recipes on your skin is going to offer a much more natural and healthier option of treatment that will help to heal your skin in no time.

Essential oils have been used for helping to improve the health and well-being of humans in mind, body and spirit throughout history. Essential oils can be used to heal wounds, reduce scarring, stretch marks, repair damage to skin due to aging, reduce inflammation, and bacterial infections just to name a few things they can help to treat. I hope that you will enjoy using my collection of essential oil recipes for skin treatments.

Chapter 1. Essential Oils

Humans have made use of wonderful essential oils to help improve different areas in our lives. We have made use of the remarkable essential oils and their benefits for centuries, they have helped us with healing wounds to repairing skin damage due to aging and everything in between. You can purchase products that have essential oils in them or you can choose to make your own homemade products with essential oils.

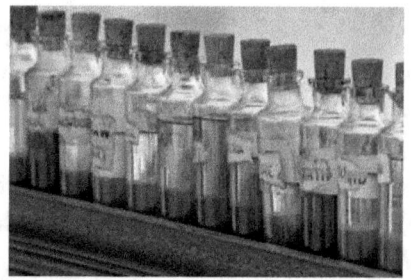

When using essential oils, it is vital that you use them with care to avoid injury. Essential oils are highly concentrated so most applications using them involve the use of carrier oils such as olive oil, coconut and almond oil amongst others. You must never directly apply essential oils to your skin or mucous membranes. Also keep in mind that essential oils do not dilute in water and must be diluted with a carrier oil. The carrier oils will also often offer their own natural benefits to your skin.

- Jojoba oil is an emollient and conditioner that offers UV protection
- Coconut oil is an antioxidant with emollient and conditioning properties.
- Rosehip seed oil helps to reduce scars, age spots and rejuvenates cells.
- Sunflower seed oil is an emollient, conditioner and skin protector.
- Olive oil provides an excellent all-around skin care: it heals, its an emollient, it protects and nourishes.

To ensure the best quality in carrier oils use oils that are organic, unrefined, and expeller-pressed, this will help to ensure you will get the best results.

When you want to add essential oils to carrier oils, decide what effect you want the product to have, then choose a combination of carrier oils and essential oils that will achieve the desired effect you are seeking.

Keep the following several rules of thumb in mind:

- Essential oils when in their concentrated state should not come into contact with skin or mucous membranes.
- Never add undiluted essential oils to you bath water. Add them first to bath salts or bath oil, then add them add to bathwater.
- When using citrus oils these can cause sun sensitivities for 12 to 24 hours after application.
- Do a patch test by applying a small amount of diluted essential oil on the skin of your inner elbow to see if you are at risk of an allergy.
- In case you are sensitive or have a reaction, flush with vegetable oil not water.
- Do not use essential oils when you are pregnant or breastfeeding.

Make sure to choose quality essential oils, rather than synthetic. You are more likely to have an allergic reaction to inferior quality essential oils. A good indication of the quality of the essential oil is the price of it. You should expect to pay between $25 to $50 for an ounce of it. Look on the label of bottle for key-words such as genuine, pure, natural, authentic, complete, not redistilled.

- "Genuine" and "authentic" essential oils are produced using a water/steam distillation; they are not dry-steam distilled.
- "Pure" essential oils are oils that contain no other essential oils or vegetable oils.
- "Natural" means that no synthetic ingredients were added to the essential oil.

- "Complete" means that the essential oil has not been modified in any way from its natural state.

Store essential oils away or out of reach of children, making sure that the lids are securely closed, in a cool, dark place.

The most common method of distillation is where water or steam is used to extract the essence. Other methods to procure the essential oils include: expression, which is referred to as cold-pressing, which is typically used with citrus oils by soaking the zest or rind in warm water and pressing it until the water and oil are pressed out of it.

Another type of distillation is solvent extraction, where another material is used such as ethyl alcohol to release the oil from the plant. The solvent extraction method is most often used when extracting more delicate flora. It is very important that the solvent used is of excellent quality as this will directly affect the purity level of the essential oil.

Essential oils are used often in perfumes, soaps, and cosmetics. They are also used in food and drink for flavoring, and even in household cleaning products. Historically, essential oils were used medicinally, although here in modern times more and more people are starting to turn to using alternative medicines over pharmaceutical synthetic products such as essential oil based treatments. Essential oils can address multiple issues due to their "adaptogenic" nature and their ability to adapt to the situation the human body is facing. Our bodies know how and where to use the compounds found in essential oils to support our needs—even if we are not aware of what our needs are!

When it comes to essential oils they are labeled "GRAS" (generally regarded as safe). Much of the danger associated with essential oils is relative to the grade of purity of the essential oil. If the brand of essential oil has been designated for aromatherapy use only, that oil should not be used for any other purpose as allergic reactions could develop along with the occurrence of toxic build up over time.

You might be wondering how can they be deemed as safe to use if there is toxicity as a factor. Toxicity becomes a factor when synthetic means are used to extract the essential oils or other non-essential oils are mixed with them. There are companies that claim that their essential oils are 100% pure, but this is why it is important that you read the fine print on the bottles. The bottle might only contain 5% percent of pure essential oil and the rest is non-essential oil ingredients. This is another reason why the grade of the essential oil is important.

Essential oils are 50-70x more powerful than their herbal complement. Check to see what type of containers the essential oil is housed in. Essential oils can pull toxic chemicals out of plastics and rubbers, these toxins will taint the contents of the container. Do not store essential oils in plastic or rubber containers to avoid contamination. Store in dark glass containers.

Quality of Essential Oils

You might be wondering why the quality of your essential oils matters, since there is no standardized industry measures out there. A bottle of essential oil only needs to contain 5-10% of actual essential oil in order to label itself as pure.

This is why you can buy over the counter essential oils for really cheap. Carrier oils are used to fill up the rest of the bottle. Synthetic oils are often used to increase the amount of oil in the bottle, these are man made compounds that mimic essential oils. Other impurities that come when the plants are harvested such as pesticides or fertilizers, the quality of the soil, air and extraction processes are some of the things that can influence the purity and quality of the essential oils being harvested. Below are basic gradations, or levels of quality, that can help you to decide what types of oils are best suited for your needs.

1. **Floral Water**—This is a by-product of the distillation process, it can possess high quality if the base materials used are organically sourced and distilled using uncompromised methods.

2. **Perfume Grade**—This grade often contains synthetics and carrier oils as well as solvents (chemicals that are used to harvest oils).

3. **Food Grade**—This grade of essential oil could contain pesticides and fertilizers (the amount will depend on where and how the crop was grown). Will contain synthetics and carrier oils.

4. **Therapeutic Grade**—This grade is made from organic sources and uses more holistic harvesting methods such as steam distillation or expression (meaning, cold pressed).

It also matters where the plant was grown, part of the plant that was used, type of extraction and how the plants were grown (wild-crafted, organic, or traditional).

Essential Oils and Helping to Manage Mood

Because of the powerful compounds in essential oils there is a wide spectrum of these oils that can be used to help us to manage our moods and emotions so that we may achieve balance in our lives. There are essential oils that can help to mitigate emotions such as anxiety, and help to bring us to a calm state.

In our microwave society, we have been primed to accept that healing comes by addressing symptoms and then this causes them to cease. We are made to believe that all pain should stop immediately. Pain in general is looked upon as a bad thing. However, without pain, we would not be aware that something was wrong. If we are not aware that something is wrong then we cannot properly treat it or address it. So, pain actually does serve a very important purpose.

The natural approach to healing can look or seem a lot different from the approach we were raised to know. In order for us to receive balance in life, we must let go of old patterns. Essential oils can be used to help bring supressed emotions to the surface. This can help us to take an honest look at what is happening within us. The essential oils will not do the emotional work for us but they can help us to prepare to release old patterns with much greater ease, if we are willing to do so.

Essential oils directly affect the limbic system when they are used aromatically. The limbic system houses several structures in our brains that affect emotion and mood. Due to bio-chemicals being released into our systems this causes us to experience emotions. The interactions that essential oils and these bio-chemical compounds have can help to shift our mood.

Application of Essential Oils

Aromatically:

Steaming: 3 to 6 drops in a cup of hot water for steam diffusing (keep your eyes closed).

Diffusing: You can purchase diffusers that come in all kinds of shapes and sizes, or you can use a simplistic method such as adding a few drops of essential oil to a tissue and breathing it in as needed. If you want to cover a large area then I would suggest using a diffuser.

Spritzing: 10-12 drops per ounce, shake well. Use a glass bottle not plastic.

Topically:

Some essential oils can be used neat, or without a carrier oil (like Melaleuca and lavender). Most essential oils will need a carrier oil for effective application. Below is a table of ratios to get you started:

For Children:

.5-1% dilution or 3-6 drops per 1 ounce of carrier oil

For Adults:

2.5% dilution or 15 drops per 1 ounce of carrier oil

3% dilution or 20 drops per 1 ounce of carrier oil

5% dilution or 30 drops per 1 ounce of carrier oil

10% dilution or 60 drops per 1 ounce of carrier oil

Internally:

Certain therapeutic grade essential oils can be taken internally in small quantities. It is very important that you do your research before using essential oils.

Chapter 2. Essential Oils Vs. Pharmaceuticals

The cells in the human body are hydrophobic, which means that they repel water. This is why your physician does not give you antibiotics when you have a viral infection, due to the fact that antibiotics are water based and can only attack the bacteria that live on the outside of the cell. Essential oils on the other hand, have the amazing ability to cross the membrane and enter the cell, and are able to promote health from the inside out. Essential oils can even cross the blood brain barrier!

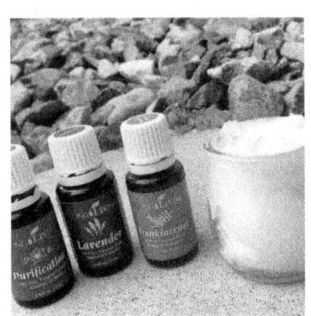

It is important to highlight some of differences between essential oils and pharmaceuticals in terms of how our health can be supported. In standard western medical treatments pharmaceuticals are the common treatment used. A reductionist point of view is what is taken from this system, treating only the symptoms associated with it. For example, if you have an allergy you will be given something to control the symptoms that accompany your allergy. The cause of those symptoms may not be directly addressed. On the other hand, with a structuralistic point of view, the whole system is considered. For example, not only will the symptoms of the allergy be looked at, but also the types of foods an individual is consuming, home environment, amount of sleep etc. will be brought into consideration. Essential oils can be viewed as an assistant to structural approaches in supporting your overall health.

Essential Oils	Pharmaceuticals
Natural	**Synthetically Engineered**
-Contain multiple naturally	-Contain 1 to 2 active ingredients

Occurring chemical compounds

-Not patentable	-Are patented
-Improves cellular functioning	-Breaks cellular communication
-No negative side effects	-Side effects that range from mild to severe
-Builds immune system	-Depresses immune system
-Adaptogenic/Wide spectrum	-Limited spectrum
-Supports the body so it can heal	-Addresses only presenting symptoms

Chapter 3. Collection of Essential Oil Based Skin and Hair Treatments

1. Wood Violet (Viola odorata)
Treatment for Dull and Tired Skin:

In your daily day cream dilute 1 drop of wood violet essential oil and apply it to your face, avoiding around the eye area.

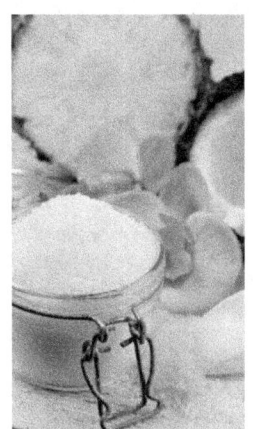

2. Bitter Orange (Citrus aurantium)
Treatment for Dull Skin:

In your day cream add in 1 drop of orange essential oil. Add to a drop of cream that is about the size of a hazelnut. Blend and apply to your skin, avoiding area around your eyes.

For Mature Skin:

Dilute 15 drops of bitter orange essential oil and 15 drops of rosewood essential oil in 100ml of Argan oil. Blend well. Apply a few drops daily, in the evening. After you have applied this treatment do not expose your skin to the sun for two hours, because this essential oil is photosensitizing.

3. Atlas Cedar (Cedar atlantica)
Treatment for Oily Hair and Hair Loss:

Dilute 4-5 drops of atlas cedar essential oil in your daily dose of shampoo and massage it lightly into your scalp. Do not use this essential oil on fragile or dry hair. It can treat oily or receding hair.

4. Cade Juniper (Juniperus oxycedrus)
Treatment for Dull Hair:

Dilute 3 drops of cade juniper essential oil in a glass container along with 10ml of sweet almond oil. Apply this blend with your hair before you wash it, massage into scalp in circular motions. Leave it in for 30 minutes, then rinse and apply shampoo. It will strengthen your hair giving it shine and lustre.

5. Roman chamomile (Chamaemelu m nobile)
Treatment to Help Soothe Irritated Skin:

Add 1-2 drops of roman chamomile essential oil to your container of hydrating cream.

6. Niaouli (melaleuca quinquen-ervia)
Treatment for Dull Tired Skin:

Add 1 drop of niaouli essential oil to a small amount of your day cream (size of a hazelnut) and apply it to your skin, avoid areas around your eyes.

7. Tea Tree (Melaleuca alternifolia)
Treatment for Acne:

After cleansing your face, apply 1 drop of tea tree oil to each pimple.

For Oily Hair:

Pour 1-2 drops of tea tree essential oil in your dose of shampoo. Shampoo your hair and avoid eyes.

8. Helichrysum (Helichrysum)
Treatment for Rosacea:

Add 10 drops of this essential oil to 100ml of your day cream. Apply this daily to your clean face.

9. Laudanum (Cistus ladaniferus)
Treatment for Acne and Pimples:

Pour 4-5 drops of laudanum essential oil into a bowl of hot water. Hold your face over the bowl of water. Remain like this for 2 minutes.

For Rosacea and Wrinkles:

Add 1 drop of laudanum essential oil to your day cream. Apply to the skin avoiding eye area.

10. Wild Carrot (daucus carota)
Treatment for Acne, Dull skin, Age Spots, and Wrinkles:

This oil will lighten skin, tighten it and accelerate healing. It is suitable for dry, combination or oily skin.

For Rosacea:

Add 1 drop of wild carrot essential oil to a small amount of your day cream (size of hazelnut) and apply it to your face making sure to avoid area around your eyes.

For Acne:

Apply 1 drop of pure wild carrot essential oil to pimples, in the morning and again in the evening.

Reduce Wrinkles and Sagging Skin:

In a glass container mix 40 drops of wild carrot essential oil and 150ml of rosehip oil. In the morning and again in the evening apply this mixture to problem areas.

11. Lovage (Levisticum officinale)
Treatment for Psoriasis:

Dilute 3 drops of lovage essential oil in a teaspoon of vegetable oil and apply to the affected areas. Do not expose yourself to the sun for the next two hours after applying, because this essential oil is photosensitizing.

12. Holy Basil (Ocimum sanctum)
Treatment for Mature, Tired, Dull Skin:

It is not suitable for people with sensitive skin. Apply 1 drop of holy basil essential oil to your usual dose of day cream and massage into your skin, avoiding areas around eyes.

13. Mandarin (citrus reticulata var. mandarin)
Treatment to Reduce Cellulite:

Blend 3-4 drops of mandarin essential oil with 1 tablespoon of macadamia oil. In the mornings and again in the evenings massage into the affected areas.

14. Sweet Fennel (Foeniculum vulgare var. Dulce)
Treatment to Help Reduce Cellulite:

Mix 40 drops of sweet fennel essential oil with 100ml of vegetable oil, along with 30 drops of grapefruit essential oil. Use this blend every night on problem areas, massaging it into them.

15. Ginger (Zingiber officinalis)
Treatment to Help Combat Hair Loss:

Add 2 drops of ginger essential oil to your daily dose of shampoo, massage it into your scalp lightly. Keep it away from your eyes. Leave blend in for 3 minutes then rinse.

16. Ylang-Ylang (Cananga odorata)
Treatment to Help Slow Down Hair Loss:

Add 1 drop of ylang-ylang essential oil to your daily dose of shampoo. If you have dry hair add 1 tablespoon of Argan oil and 1 drop of this essential oil to your scalp and massage it lightly into your hair. Leave it on for 1 minute, rinse and apply shampoo with drop of ylang-ylang essential oil.

17. Rosemary camphor (Rosmarinus officinalis cam-phoriferum)
Relaxing Foot Bath:

Not recommended for people with epilepsy. Dilute 5 drops of rosemary camphor essential oil in 1 tablespoon of vegetable oil and a handful of coarse salt. Pour into a bowl filled with warm water and immerse your feet into the mixture for 10 minutes.

To Reduce Cellulite:

Dilute 1 drop of rosemary camphor essential oil and 1 drop of grapefruit essential oil in 1 tablespoon of sweet almond oil. Apply it in the morning and in the evening on buttocks, thighs and stomach, massaging problem areas.

18. Patchouli (Pogostemon cablin)
Treatment for Minor Skin Irritations Such as Eczema and Acne:

Dilute 3 drops of patchouli essential oil in 1 teaspoon of rosehip oil and apply to problem area.

19. Lemon verbena (Lippia citriodora)
Treatment for Cleaning Clogged Pores, and Purifying Oily Skin:

Pour 5 drops of lemon verbena essential oil into a bowl of hot water. Hold your face above the bowl of water, and cover head with a towel. Stay like this for 2 minutes and then wipe your face with a face cloth. Do not expose yourself to the sun for the next 2 hours after treatment, because this essential oil is photosensitizing.

20. Grapefruit (Citrus paradisii)
Treatment for Tightening skin, and Helps to Prevent Sagging in Skin. It is also helpful for oily skin. It can also be used as a prophylactic treatment against cellulite.

For Oily Skin:

Pour 3-4 drops of grapefruit essential oil into a bowl of hot water and hold your face above the bowl. Cover your head with a towel, close your eyes and stay like this for 2 minutes. Remove excess oil with a cotton ball.

For Cellulite:

Dilute 5 drops of grapefruit essential oil in 2 tablespoons of jojoba oil and massage into your buttocks, stomach, and thighs. After this treatment do not expose yourself to the sun for two hours, because this essential oil is photosensitizing.

21. Lime (citrus aurantifolia)
Treatment for Lightening Complexion and Treating Oily Skin:

For Oily Skin:

Make a facial mask with 2 tablespoons of green clay and 1 tablespoon of hazelnut oil and 1 drop of lime essential oil. Add a little bit of water and mix until you have a thick paste. Apply the paste to your face, avoiding areas around your eyes. Let the mask rest for 10 minutes, then rinse. Do not expose yourself to the sun for two hours after this treatment, because the essential oil is photosensitizing.

22. Lemon (citrus limonum)
For Treatment of Oily Skin:

Dilute 1 drop of lemon essential oil in 1 teaspoon of hazelnut oil and apply to your face.

For Treatment to Reduce Cellulite:

Mix 3 drops of lemon essential oil with 1 tablespoon of vegetable oil and apply it to problem areas daily, massaging into the skin.

For Treatment of Dandruff:

Add 2 drops of lemon essential oil to your daily dose of shampoo.

23. Damask rose (Rosa damascena)

This essential oil works great in the treatment of tired skin, wrinkles, dull skin and also promotes healing.

Treatment for Aging Skin:

Add 1 drop of damask rose essential oil to your day cream (100ml). Blend well, with a small spatula. Apply this cream in the day to clean and dry face.

Treatment for Dull, Tired Skin:

Dilute 4 drops of damask rose essential oil and 2 drops of rosewood essential oil in 75ml of rosehip oil. Apply a few drops of this blend, before bedtime, to clean skin.

24. Neroli (Citrus aurantium)

This essential oil is good to use on sensitive skin, mature skin and rosacea.

Treatment to Help Reduce Wrinkles:

Add 1 drop of neroli essential oil to a small amount of your day cream (size of hazelnut) and apply it to your skin. Avoid areas around your eyes.

25. Myrtle Green (Myrtus communis cineoliferum)
Treatment to Smooth Out Wrinkles:

Add 1 drop of myrtle green essential oil to a small amount of your day cream (size of hazelnut), and apply it to your skin. Make sure to avoid areas around your eyes.

26. Lemon Balm (Melissa officinalis)
This essential oil has anti-aging properties and helps to fight against premature aging.

Treatment to Fight Against Premature Aging:

Add 1 drop of lemon balm essential oil to your usual dose of day cream and massage into your skin, avoid areas around your eyes.

27. Jasmine (Jasminum grandiflorum)
Treatment for Reducing Fine Lines, Calming Acne, and Accelerate Healing:

Dilute 1 drop of jasmine essential oil in 1 tablespoon of vegetable oil and add this blend into your bath water. Enjoy the wonderful scent of jasmine, it will help you to relax too! You can also wear this essential oil as a perfume. Apply one drop behind your earlobe and you are all set!

28. Turmeric (Curcuma longa)
Treatment for Wrinkles and Fine Lines:

Dilute 5 drops of turmeric essential oil in 10ml of borage seed oil. Apply a few drops of blend each morning, to a clean face, avoiding areas around your eyes.

29. Geranium Rosat (pelargonium asperum)
Geranium Rosat essential oil will help against wrinkles, age spots, sagging skin, hair loss, and acne. It can also help to remove cellulite.

Treatment to Prevent Stretch Marks:

Mix 15 drops of geranium rosat essential oil with 50ml of borage seed oil. Apply this blend in the mornings and evenings on your buttocks, thighs and stomach.

Treatment to Prevent Wrinkles:

Mix 8 drops of geranium rosat essential oil, 8 drops of rosewood essential oil, with 50ml of evening primrose oil in a glass container. Apply this blend in gentle circular motions, after you have removed your makeup.

Treatment Against Hair Loss:

Add 2 drops of geranium rosat essential oil to your daily dose of shampoo and massage it into your scalp lightly then rinse.

30. Tansy (tanacetum annuum)
Tansy essential oil is not recommended for people with epilepsy. This essential oil is often used to soothe skin suffering from sunburn, dermatitis, and eczema. It can help to reduce minor inflammation.

Treatment of Skin Irritations:

Dilute 2 drops of tansy essential oil in a few drops of sweet almond oil or rosehip oil and apply gently to affected area.

Chapter 4. Bonus Recipe Collection!

31. Vanilla (vanilla planifolia)
Vanilla essential oil works great at helping to hydrate and regenerate your skin.

Treatment for Hydrating Skin:

Add a drop of vanilla essential oil to your daily dose of day cream and apply it to your skin, avoiding areas around your eyes. You can also add 15 drops of vanilla essential oil to your shower gel (right into the bottle) to give it a lovely scent.

32. Frankincense or Olibanum (boswellia carterii)
Frankincense essential oil has strengthening and regenerative properties. It also helps to soothe and soften dry skin.

Treatment for Dry Skin:

Add 1 drop of Frankincense essential oil to a small amount of your day cream (about size of hazelnut) and massage into skin, avoiding areas around your eyes.

33. Garden Angelica (Angelica archangelica)
Treatment for Soothing and Softening Dry Skin:

Add 1 drop of garden angelica essential oil to your daily dose of day cream, and apply to skin, avoiding areas around your eyes. Do not expose yourself to the sun for two hours after this treatment, because this essential oil is photosensitizing.

34. Essential Oil Blend Body Powder

If you want to normalize your skin and feel refreshed and comfortable all day, then this might be a recipe that you should consider trying.

Ingredients:

- 10 drops of spruce essential oil
- 10 drops of peppermint essential oil
- 5 drops of clove essential oil
- 2 tablespoons of corn starch
- 2 tablespoons of spearmint

35. Natural and Pure Skin Toner

Do you suffer from pigmentation or do you have dark age spots that you would like to get rid of? Why not try this blend of lavender, Palmarosa and rosewood essential oils? This mix will give you a gentle toning effect that will help you to get rid of some of your skin imperfections within a few days. You can spray this essential oil blend onto your skin or you can rub it on to your skin using your hands.

Ingredients:

- 2 drops of lavender essential oil
- 1 drop of Palmarosa essential oil
- 1 drop of rosewood essential oil
- 8 ounces of distilled water

36. Essential Oil Treatment for Psoriasis:

Psoriasis is a hair disorder that can be painful and very difficult to handle for many that suffer from it. Essential oils such as tea tree and sage essential oils can help to get rid of this problem gradually because of the powerful antiseptic and antibacterial properties that they have. The essential oils will also help to stimulate healing of the scalp from within. Plants such as sage can help clarify the scalp and open it up for penetration of the healing substances within the essential oils.

Ingredients:

- 4 drops of sage essential oil
- 3 drops of tea tree essential oil
- 2 drops rosemary essential oil
- 2 tablespoons of sweet almond oil

Directions:

Blend all of the oils in a small bowl together and then apply mix to scalp. Massage into scalp leaving on for 10 minutes, then rinse.

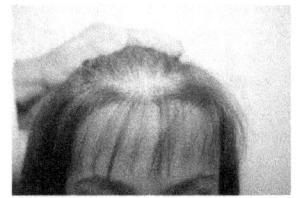

37. Recipe for Treating Oily Hair:

Oily hair is always messy looking and dirt can get easily stuck in it, it can be a real challenge to clean. Essential oils such as Patchouli essential oil help to reduce oils in your hair by as much as 60% and will also help to stimulate hair regrowth.

Ingredients:

- 3 drops lemongrass essential oil
- 2 drops Patchouli essential oil
- 2 drops Rosemary essential oil

Directions:

Add the essential oils to your shampoo and blend. Massage into your scalp lightly and leave on for a few minutes, then rinse.

38. Essential Oil Blend for Treating Dandruff

Do you have a sore scalp or are you noticing that you are losing your hair due to dandruff? Essential oils such as cedarwood, and clary sage have been shown in clinical studies to help clear issues on the scalp.

Ingredients:

- 3 drops of clary sage essential oil
- 3 drops of cedarwood essential oil
- 2 drops of chamomile essential oil
- 2 drops of Eucalyptus essential oil

Directions:

Add the above essential oils to your regular shampoo and apply to your scalp massaging gently into scalp. Leave on for 5 minutes then rinse. Avoid getting in eyes.

39. Dull Skin Essential Oil Treatment

Using a mix of clove with cinnamon and orange essential oils can help to rejuvenate dry skin and make it supple in a few minutes. Clove has powerful antioxidants in it that will destroy oxidative stress on the skin, while the wild orange essential oil will help to purify skin pores.

Ingredients:

- 2 drops wild orange essential oil
- 2 drops cinnamon essential oil
- 2 drops clove essential oil

Directions:

Add these essential oils to your daily day cream and apply to your skin. Use day cream of at least the same size of a hazelnut. Avoid contact with your eyes.

40. Skin Softening and Healing Recipe

Dilute the following essential oil mix into your bath and enjoy the aromatherapy power of these skin rejuvenating essential oils!

Ingredients:

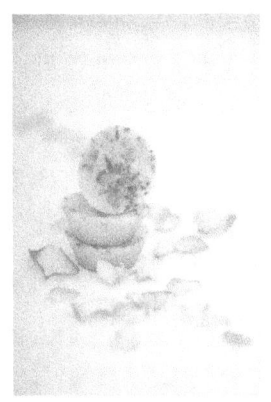

- 8-10 drops lavender essential oil
- 2-3 drops Palmarosa essential oil
- 2-3 drops Rose essential oil
- 2-3 drops Geranium essential oil

41. Muscle Relief Essential Oil Massage

The oils that are used in this recipe work great for helping to relieve tired muscles, especially those suffering from arthritis and poor circulation. The best way to use this is to massage it into your muscles after a warm bath or shower.

Ingredients:

- 15 drops of juniper essential oil
- 15 drops of marjoram essential oil
- 10 drops of rosemary essential oil
- 5 drops of black pepper essential oil
- 3 tablespoons of grapeseed oil

Directions:

Blend all of the oils in a glass container, and apply to area of sore muscles.

42. Essential Oil Massage for Over Exerted Muscles:

This wonderful essential oil blend works great for helping to relax those overused muscles. Massage this blend into your tired muscles after you have had a warm bath or shower.

Ingredients:

- 5 drops of eucalyptus essential oil
- 5 drops of ginger essential oil
- 5 drops of peppermint essential oil
- 1 tablespoon of sweet almond oil

Directions:

Blend all of your oil in a glass bowl, and apply onto your sore muscles massaging into them.

43. Essential Oil Blend for Muscle Cramps:
This blend is great if you are suffering from muscle cramps. The best way to use this is to apply after you have had a warm bath or shower.

Ingredients:

- 5 drops lavender essential oil
- 5 drops rosemary essential oil
- 5 drops marjoram essential oil
- 3 drops of black pepper essential oil
- 5 teaspoons of coconut oil

Directions:

This muscle soak will be a great addition to your warm bath or shower when you are looking for a way to relax your sore muscles.

44. Simple Bruise Oil:
Using this oil blend will help to reduce the appearance of bruising by helping to promote circulation and healing the damaged tissue. Gently massage this oil blend onto bruised skin.

Ingredients:

- 2 drops rosemary essential oil
- 2 drops geranium essential oil
- 1 drop lavender essential oil
- 1 teaspoon jojoba oil

Directions:

Blend all of your oils in a glass container, and apply the oil blend gently on the bruised skin.

45. Massage Oil for Rheumatism:

This blend of essential oils is for those who suffer from rheumatoid arthritis and are looking for a safe and effective way to soothe their sore joints. Use this treatment after you have had a warm shower or bath.

Ingredients:

- 4 drops cypress essential oil
- 2 drops juniper essential oil
- 2 drops roman chamomile essential oil
- 3 drops rosemary essential oil
- 4 teaspoons of sweet almond oil

Directions:

Blend these oils in a glass container, then apply onto area where needed.

46. Body Butter for Varicose Veins:

This body butter is a great option to help treat the effects of varicose veins. To prepare this recipe you will use a double broiler over medium-low heat, stirring the Shea butter and coconut oil for a few minutes until it melts. Once it has melted, remove it from heat and add in the rest of your ingredients. Place it in the fridge for an hour. After an hour, remove from fridge and mix it with hand mixer for ten minutes or until soft peaks are formed. You 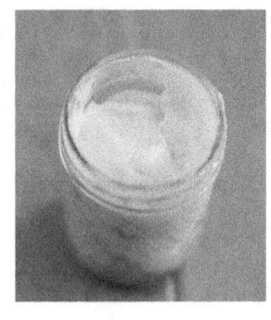 can store it in a glass container for up to six months. Use blend daily in the mornings.

Ingredients:

- 5 drops of cypress essential oil
- 10 drops of Helichrysum essential oil
- 10 drops of fennel essential oil
- 5 drops of lemon essential oil
- ½ cup of Shea butter
- ¼ cup of coconut oil
- ¼ cup of jojoba oil

Directions:

Heat Shea butter and coconut oil in double broiler over medium-low heat. Once the butter and oil has melted stir and blend and remove from heat. Allow to cool down then add into glass container along with remaining ingredients and blend well. Place in fridge for an hour, then remove and blend with hand blender until it forms into peaks. It can be stored in glass container up to six months. Use daily in the mornings.

47. Body Scrub for Sensitive Skin:
Ingredients:

- 4 drops lavender essential oil
- 3 drops geranium essential oil
- 3 drops roman chamomile essential oil
- ¼ cup of coconut oil
- 1 ½ cups of sea salt

Directions:

Mix ingredients of body scrub in a bowl together. Apply scrub on damp skin, and then rub over skin. Rinse off skin.

48. Body Scrub for Oily Skin:
Ingredients:

- 5 drops of rosemary essential oil
- 5 drops of tea tree essential oil
- 1 ½ cups of ground coffee
- ¼ cup of jojoba oil

Directions:

Blend ingredients in a glass container, and apply to skin. Rub over skin. Rinse off.

49. Body Scrub for Skin with Eczema
Ingredients:

- 4 drops lavender essential oil
- 3 drops neroli essential oil
- 3 drops carrot seed essential oil
- 1 ½ cups of sugar

- ¼ cup of olive oil

Directions:

Blend all of your ingredients in a glass bowl, then apply to affected areas of skin. Rub over skin and then rinse off.

50. Stretch Mark Serum:

This serum will help to provide nourishment, and hydration, as well as fading and preventing stretch marks, rebuilding collagen, increasing circulation and elasticity of your skin. Use this serum once or twice a day to reduce the appearance of stretch marks and scars.

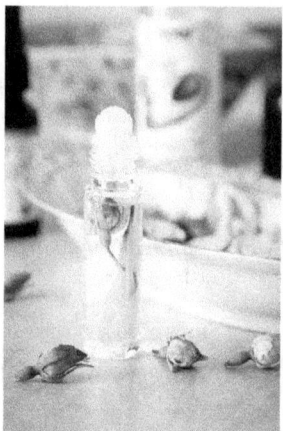

Ingredients:

- 5 drops myrrh essential oil
- 5 drops lavender essential oil
- 5 drops neroli essential oil
- 5 drops lemon essential oil
- 2 tablespoons of rosehip oil
- 2 tablespoons of jojoba oil
- 2 tablespoons of vitamin E oil

Directions:

Blend all of your ingredients well in a glass container, then apply to affected area of skin.

Conclusion

I hope that you and your loved ones will enjoy using this collection of essential oil based recipes that focus mainly on treating minor skin conditions. I am sure you will feel good in knowing that these recipes do not have any synthetic chemicals included in them. You will really begin to see how much your skin enjoys these natural remedies when you see your healthy glowing skin after you begin to use them. These natural products are not only a healthy option but they will also save you a lot of money making them yourself compared to purchasing products at the shops.

I wish to thank you once again for downloading my book, and supporting my work. It is very much appreciated, I hope to read a review of my book by you on Amazon.

FREE Bonus Reminder

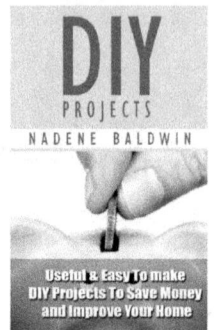

If you have not grabbed it yet, please go ahead and download your special bonus report *"DIY Projects. 13 Useful & Easy To Make DIY Projects To Save Money & Improve Your Home!"*

Simply Click the Button Below

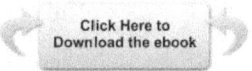

OR **Go to This Page**

http://diyhomecraft.com/free

BONUS #2: More Free & Discounted Books or Products

Do you want to receive more Free/Discounted Books or Products?

We have a mailing list where we send out our new Books or Products when they go free or with a discount on Amazon. Click on the link below to sign up for Free & Discount Book & Product Promotions.

=> Sign Up for Free & Discount Book & Product Promotions <=

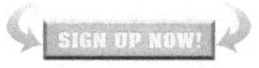

OR Go to this URL

http://zbit.ly/1WBb1Ek

www.ingramcontent.com/pod-product-compliance
Lightning Source LLC
Chambersburg PA
CBHW061934280526
45787CB00004B/1597